# Otolaryngologic Examination

*Toronto Physical Examination Series*
*General Editor: Donald L. Levene, M.D.*

# E.N.T.

## Otolaryngologic Examination

**J. M. Nedzelski, M.D.**
University of Toronto
Sunnybrook Medical Centre, Toronto

Collier Macmillan Canada, Ltd.

Collier Macmillan Canada, Ltd.
1125B Leslie Street, Don Mills, Ontario M3C 2K2

ISBN 02-991390-X

Design: Michael van Elsen

Illustrations by Jackie Heda, B.S., Department of Art as
Applied to Medicine, University of Toronto

1 2 3 4 5 6 84 83 82 81 80

Printed and bound in Canada


Canadian Cataloguing in Publication Data

Nedzelski, J.M., 1943 –
    E.N.T. : otolaryngologic examination

(Toronto physical examination series)

ISBN 0-02-991390-X

1. Otolaryngologic examination – Handbooks, manuals, etc.
I. Title.  II. Title: Otolaryngologic examination.  III. Series.

RF48.N42   617′.51   C80-094319-8

# Contents

# Head Mirror

DO'S

– the back of the mirror almost touches the forehead, cheek

– bright light source beside the patient on the examiner's mirror eye side

DONT'S

– move your own head once the light spot is focused, rather than move the patient's head (focal length fixed)

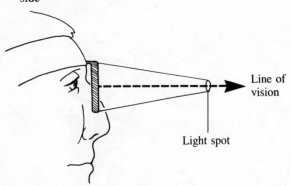

Line of vision

Light spot

– focus mirror to obtain a small bright spot

7

# External Ear

DO'S

- inspect the auricle for any abnormality
- pull the auricle up and back
- displace the tragus anteriorly
- inspect the external canal

DONT'S

- pull the auricle towards self

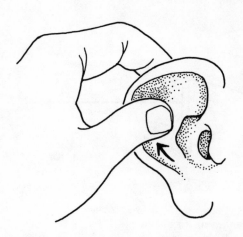

# External Auditory Canal

DO'S

- retract the auricle postero-superiorly between the middle and ring fingers

DONT'S

- insert the tip of the aural speculum beyond the cartilaginous external canal (outer ⅓) ouch!!

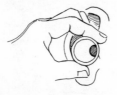

- under direct vision, gently remove cerumen and debris

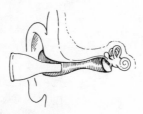

- inspect the entire drum by moving the speculum tip

# Tympanic Membrane

DESCRIPTION:
INTACT?
COLOUR?
CONTOUR?
MOBILITY?

Quadrants of pars tensa
(right drum)

Postero-superior

Antero-superior

Postero-inferior

Antero-inferior

Right tympanic membrane

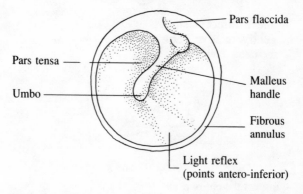

Pars flaccida

Pars tensa

Umbo

Malleus handle

Fibrous annulus

Light reflex
(points antero-inferior)

Use otoscope to supplement speculum for detailed examination of the drumhead

10

INTACT?

Perforation
central (drum margin = annulus present)

marginal (annulus absent)

central
(safe)

marginal attic
(potentially unsafe
due to skin migration
into middle ear
= cholesteatoma)

subtotal
(safe because
skin rarely
extends into middle
ear with annulus
present)

COLOUR?

red (injected)        yellow        chalky areas

acute otitis
media

serous otitis
media

tympanosclerotic
plaques

11

**CONTOUR?**

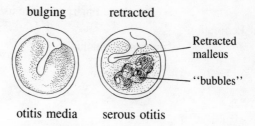

bulging     retracted

Retracted malleus

"bubbles"

otitis media     serous otitis

**MOBILITY?**

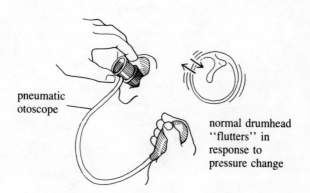

pneumatic otoscope

normal drumhead "flutters" in response to pressure change

# Describe Tympanic Membrane

INTACT?
- perforation
  - central
  - marginal
    desquamating epithelium in middle ear
    = cholesteatoma

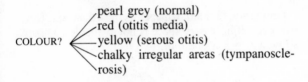

COLOUR?
- pearl grey (normal)
- red (otitis media)
- yellow (serous otitis)
- chalky irregular areas (tympanoscle-rosis)

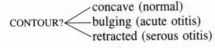

CONTOUR?
- concave (normal)
- bulging (acute otitis)
- retracted (serous otitis)

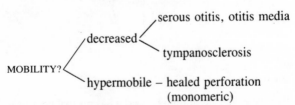

MOBILITY?
- decreased
  - serous otitis, otitis media
  - tympanosclerosis
- hypermobile – healed perforation (monomeric)

# Hearing Tests

Check the patient's ability to repeat words spoken in a whispered voice. Each ear should be tested individually ensuring that the patient cannot read your lips. The non-test ear is masked by having the patient continuously rustle paper opposite the external meatus.

Ordinarily, a loud whisper is heard at six feet. However, if necessary space is not available compare a low whisper at one foot, two feet, etc.

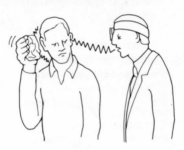

WATCH TEST

The examiner (assuming he or she has normal hearing) can compare his own ability to hear a wrist watch to that of the patient's at varying distances, i.e. six inches, twelve inches from ear.

# Tuning Fork Tests

- use a 512 Hz tuning fork

WEBER TEST
- place the stem of vibrating tuning fork in the median line of the skull, i.e. mid forehead, vertex
- ask the patient to indicate with one index finger where the sound is heard best
- in a normal individual the sound is heard equally well on both sides

Normal Weber test

- if it is heard on only one side it indicates that this ear has better bone conduction as would occur in a case of conductive type deafness or because the opposite ear has significant air conduction (sensorineural)hearing loss

RINNE TEST
- comparison of air conduction to bone conduction
- place the stem of vibrating tuning fork on the mastoid bone and ask the patient to tell you when he or she can no longer hear it
- the tuning fork is then held such that the tines are near the external meatus

15

- in patient with normal hearing or sensorineural hearing loss, the vibrating tuning fork is still heard and the test is said to be Rinne positive

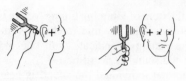

Rinne positive = AC > BC

*Note:*
- Weber lateralizes with minor conductive loss (< 5 db)
- bone conduction becomes better than air conduction (Rinne negative) only if conductive loss ≥ 20 db i.e. right conductive hearing loss

Weber                        Rinne

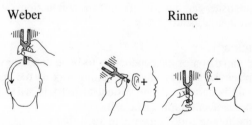

Rinne negative = BC > AC

i.e. right sensorineural hearing loss

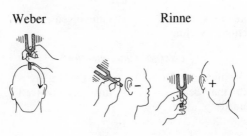

Weber                                Rinne

Rinne positive = AC > BC

i.e. right false negative Rinne test
– patient lateralizes Weber test to left ear.
– on Rinne test of right ear, patient claims that bone
  conduction (mastoid) is better than air.
– in reality, the patient is hearing bone conduction
  in the left ear – this is proven by masking the left
  ear while the Rinne is repeated on the right.

*Remember!* A vibrating fork on the mastoid stimu-
lates BOTH cochleae.

**Otitis Externa**    vs    **Otitis Media**

*auricle*

| | |
|---|---|
| severe cases: canthal injection, swelling | uninvolved |

*external canal meatus*

| | |
|---|---|
| skin swollen, tender, meatus may be occluded | skin not usually diffusely involved |

*pain*

| | |
|---|---|
| exacerbated by<br>– tragal pressure<br>– auricle displacement<br>– speculum pressing on canal walls | not changed by opposite manipulation of the external canal wall |

*tympanic membrane*

| | |
|---|---|
| – if visualized, the drum is intact and not displaced | injected, bulging if intact |

*otorrhea*

| | |
|---|---|
| thin, non-pulsating | usually thick, if pulsating in the region of the drumhead (referred from the middle ear) implies perforation |

# Ear Pain

mediated by $\begin{cases} \text{trigeminal} \\ \text{glossopharyngeal} \\ \text{vagus} \\ \text{upper cervical (}C_2, C_3\text{)} \end{cases}$

Local pain

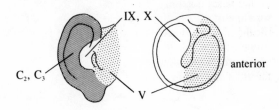

Referred pain

Ten T's

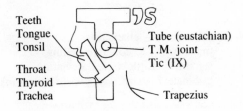

# Nasal Examination

**DO'S**

- inspect the external nose
- insert a closed speculum into the vestibule only
- rest the index finger on the nasal dorsum for support
- tilt the patient's head forward, then backward to visualize the floor and roof

**DONT'S**

- press speculum blades against the septum
- remove closed speculum from nose (ouch!!)

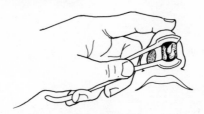

*Note:* rhinorrhea? – character
mucosa? – i.e. colour, swelling
septum? – Little's area, deviation
turbinates? – size, vasoconstrictor shrinkage

Use topical vasoconstrictor for examination

# Nasal Obstruction

nasal breathing on metal tongue depressor allows comparison of sides, semi-objective assessment

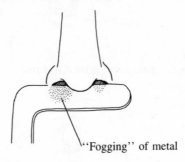

"Fogging" of metal

CONSTANT OBSTRUCTION:

Unilateral
   a) anatomic
     – deviated septum

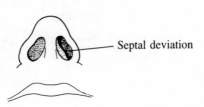

Septal deviation

– turbinate hypertrophy

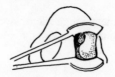

b) polyps
   – nasal – pale grey, arise nasal roof

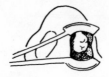

– antro-choanal polyp – arise maxillary sinus

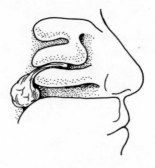

c) cancer – nasal fossa (uncommon)
   extension from sinus (more common)

BEWARE: unilateral obstruction + facial pain + blood tinged discharge = CANCER

d) foreign body – consider this in the child with intermittent unilateral mucopurulent discharge

Bilateral Obstruction
   nasal fossa – anatomic
              – polyps
   nasopharyngeal tumor
   adenoid
   cancer

INTERMITTENT OBSTRUCTION
Think of "Rhinitis" = primarily mucosal etiology
   1. Infections – viral (coryza)
                 – bacterial (associated sinusitis)
   2. Allergic – seasonal i.e. ragweed
               – dust, feathers
   3. Vasomotor (nose drips "like a tap")

# Sinuses

Examination is indirect
- palpate for tenderness over the frontal, maxillary sinuses
- examine for mucopurulent rhinorrhea in the area of the nose where draining sinus(es) are in question
- compare (left vs right) by illumination (in a totally dark room) frontal and maxillary sinuses

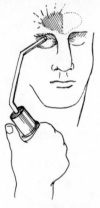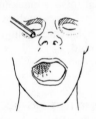

(Transillumination viewed through opened mouth)

Transillumination under the frontal sinus floor

Transillumination posterior to the infraorbital rim

# Oral Cavity and Oropharynx

DO LOOK *at*

– remove dentures if
  present
– inspect
  a) buccal mucosa
     (Stensen's duct)
     gingiva, teeth
  b) palate – hard, soft
  c) tongue (ant. ⅔)
     – inspect
     – palpate
  d) floor of mouth
     – inspect (Wharton's duct)
     – palpate (bimanual)
  e) palatine tonsils
  f) posterior pharyngeal wall

DON'T LOOK *through*

i.e. don't concentrate on
one structure eg. tonsils
at the expense of other
structures

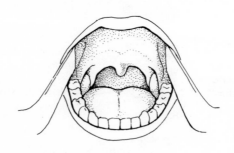

# Nasopharynx

| DO'S | DONT'S |
|---|---|
| – tongue in mouth<br>– steady tongue depression along entire dorsum<br>– ''sniffing'' effort by the patient with the mirror in place<br>– slowly tilt the mirror from side to side | – dig tongue depressor into tongue base<br>– push the mirror into the posterior pharyngeal wall |

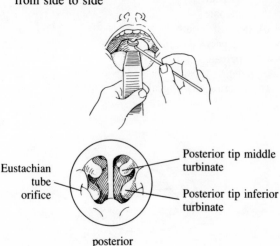

Eustachian tube orifice

Posterior tip middle turbinate

Posterior tip inferior turbinate

posterior

# Hypopharynx and Larynx

DO'S

- *hold* the protruding
  tip of the tongue in
  gauze
- support the upper lip
- have the patient
  quietly breath through
  the mouth
- elevate the uvula with
  the back of a warmed
  mirror
- inspect:
  base of tongue:
  (post. ⅓)
  larynx
  quiet respiration,
  phonating "eee"

DONT'S

- *pull* the tongue
- push the mirror
  against the
  pharyngeal wall

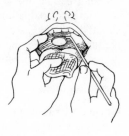

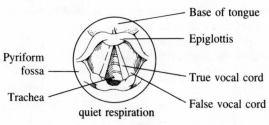

Base of tongue

Epiglottis

Pyriform fossa

True vocal cord

Trachea

False vocal cord

quiet respiration

# Neck Examination

- inspection of the neck from anterior, posterior and lateral aspects is first carried out
- detailed examination of the neck is conducted by palpation in systematic fashion. Examination technique of palpation of the neck can be done with the examiner facing the patient or with the examiner standing behind the seated patient. Remember to use bimanual palpation, move the neck structures about, have the patient turn his head laterally to facilitate getting around the strap muscles, hyperextend the neck to better assess the thyroid gland.

ANTERIOR NECK

- bimanual examination of the submental triangle with index finger of one hand in floor of patient's mouth palpating against opposite hand
- palpate the hyoid bone, thyroid cartilages, cervical trachea, noting mobility, position
- note thyroid gland position, size, shape, tenderness, mobility using bimanual palpation standing behind patient. Have the patient cough, swallow to detect possible lower pole enlargement.
- palpate the suprasternal notch

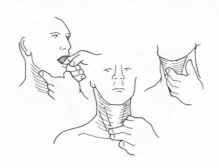

## LATERAL NECK

– bimanual palpation of the submandibular triangle is carried out noting gland size, consistency, presence of lymph nodes
– carotid bulb pulsations are noted roughly at the level of the thyroid cartilage notch
– presence of palpably enlarged cervical lymph nodes is noted
– supraclavicular fossa is checked for palpable masses

## PAROTID GLAND

– palpate the gland (normally very ill-defined) noting enlargement, consistency, tenderness, masses, overlying skin
– bimanual palpation of Stensen's duct is carried out, noting nature of secretions from duct orifice in mouth

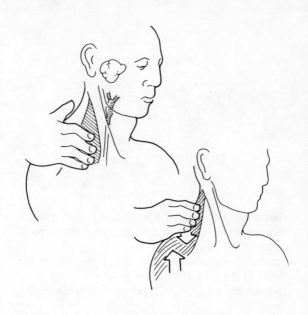

POSTEROLATERAL NECK

– palpate posterior triangle of the neck for masses
– assess function of trapezius muscle

# Neck Masses

## Midline

*Congenital*

1. Dermoid cyst
2. Thyroglossal duct cyst

*Acquired*

1. Thyroid isthmus nodule

## Lateral Neck

*Congenital*

1. Branchial cleft cysts (along anterior border of sternomastoid)

*Acquired*

1. Salivary gland tumors
2. Cervical lymph node lesion
   - lymphoreticular disease
   - metastatic disease
3. Thyroid gland lesions
   - goitre
   - nodule, etc.
4. Carotid body tumor
5. Others, i.e. neurofibroma, fibroma, lipoma
6. Zenker's diverticulum

*Remember*

A mass in the neck should be considered to be metastatic cancer from a primary carcinoma of the head and neck until proven otherwise.

# Vertigo

Vertigo – hallucination of movement of either self or environment. An accurate, detailed history is paramount in diagnosis of patients with "dizziness" or balance disturbance.

Decision tree strategy (after H. O. Barber)

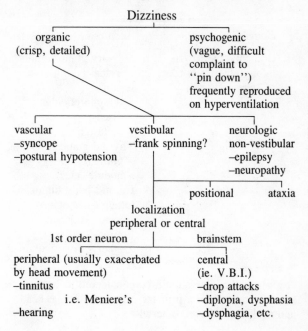

Dizziness

organic
(crisp, detailed)

psychogenic
(vague, difficult
complaint to
"pin down")
frequently reproduced
on hyperventilation

vascular
–syncope
–postural hypotension

vestibular
–frank spinning?

neurologic
non-vestibular
–epilepsy
–neuropathy

positional      ataxia

localization
peripheral or central

1st order neuron

brainstem

peripheral (usually exacerbated
by head movement)
–tinnitus
     i.e. Meniere's
–hearing

central
(ie. V.B.I.)
–drop attacks
–diplopia, dysphasia
–dysphagia, etc.

# Equilibrium Triad

1. Vestibular apparatus
2. Visual imput
3. Proprioceptive fibers of tendons, muscles, joints, especially neck.

The most important physical sign in the vertiginous patient is the presence of nystagmus.

Nystagmus – involuntary rhythmic movement of eyes about a certain axis (horizontal, rotatory, vertical) usually with alternately slow and fast phases.
Nystagmus direction is designated by that of the quick component.

Examine for:

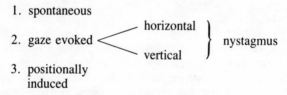

1. spontaneous

2. gaze evoked ⟨ horizontal / vertical ⟩ nystagmus

3. positionally induced

# Nystagmus

- use an easily seen small object i.e. tip of pen, small bright light which the patient can follow
- in questionable cases of nystagmus, it is helpful to fixate on a scleral vessel of the patient's eye and watch it for movement

*Note:* axis i.e. horizonal
       direction i.e. right
       amplitude i.e. coarse

SPONTANEOUS (PRIMARY GAZE POSITION) NYSTAGMUS

- have the patient look straight ahead at object eye level i.e. pen light 24″ away

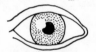 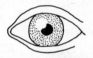

HORIZONTAL GAZE

- have the patient follow an object to the right of primary gaze positions such that gaze deviation is about 30°, then repeat to the left. Use the punctum of the lacrimal sac on the lower eyelid as a reference point; when the medial corneal margin of the adducting eye reaches a vertical line extended up from the punctum, the gaze deviation is 30°. Note: gaze deviation beyond 30° may be so-called non-pathologic end point or physiologic nystagmus.

34

Do this

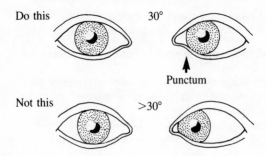

Punctum

Not this

VERTICAL GAZE

- have patient look upwards, then downwards as far
  as possible
- while having patient upgaze, elevate both eyelids
  with left hand having the patient follow the light
  source or pen held in your right hand

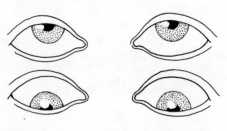

*Note:* Vertical gaze especially upgaze tends to become restricted with advancing age.

Vertical nystagmus always indicates central nervous system disease.
- upbeating nystagmus – cerebellar (anterior vermis) tumor, fourth ventricle masses, multiple sclerosis, etc.
- downbeating nystagmus – brainstem, i.e. lower medulla, upper cervical cord (Arnold Chiari)

POSITIONAL NYSTAGMUS

- screening test for positional nystagmus consists of having patient's head moved backward over edge of table in supine position with the neck twisted to one side and the position maintained for 15-30 seconds
- patient is sat up and nystagmus searched for
- test sequence repeated with head turned to opposite side

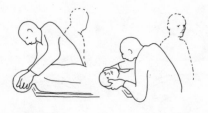

Paroxysmal Positional Nystagmus
 – noted by above maneuvre consists of
  1) rotatory nystagmus (toward undermost ear) last-
     ing less than 30 seconds
  2) patient vertiginous
  3) nystagmus onset delayed several seconds
  4) recurring in opposite direction on sitting up
  5) repeat positioning fatigues nystagmus

Paroxysmal (benign) positional nystagmus is of la-
byrinthine localization vs positional nystagmus which
is linear, persistent, direction fixed or changing with
little or no subjective vertigo indicating probable CNS
brainstem/cerebellar localization.

i.e. counterclockwise rotatory nystagmus is noted while
in head hanging right lateral position–becomes clock-
wise rotatory nystagmus after having patient sit up

**NOTES**

NOTES

# NOTES